The Anxiety Fire Drill

Your 7-Minute Plan to Stop the Spiral Before
It Starts

Robert Duane McDonald

First Edition

ISBN (Paperback): 978-1-923604-26-1

ISBN (eBook): 978-1-923604-27-8

The information provided in this book is for educational and informational purposes only and is not intended as a substitute for professional medical advice, diagnosis, or treatment. The author and publisher are not medical professionals or licensed therapists.

Always seek the advice of your physician or other qualified health provider with any questions you may have regarding a medical or mental health condition. Never disregard professional medical advice or delay in seeking it because of something you have read in this book.

If you are experiencing severe anxiety, depression, or have thoughts of self-harm, please seek immediate professional help or contact an emergency crisis hotline.

The case examples, names, characters, and incidents mentioned in this book are illustrative composites based on common experiences and are used fictitiously. Any resemblance to actual persons, living or dead, or actual events is purely coincidental. The author and publisher assume no responsibility for errors, inaccuracies, or omissions.

Table of Contents

Preface

It happens fast.

One minute you are going about your day. The next, maybe triggered by an email, a memory, or seemingly nothing at all, you feel it. The tightness in the chest. The sudden rush of heat. The heart rate that speeds up for no good reason.

This is the anxiety spiral. And when it starts, it accelerates quickly.

If you have experienced this, you know how terrifying it is. And you also know how utterly useless it is when someone tells you to "just calm down" or "try not to worry about it."

That advice fails because it misunderstands the fundamental nature of acute anxiety.

There is a biological reason why you cannot simply "think" your way out of panic. When intense anxiety hits, the part of your brain responsible for logic and rational thought—the prefrontal cortex—starts to go offline. The fear center of your brain takes over. It initiates a full-blown fight-or-flight response.

In that moment, your brain genuinely believes you are in life-threatening danger, even if you are just sitting on your couch. Trying to use logic when your survival system is activated is like trying to reason with a tornado.

If you cannot think your way out, you need a different approach. You need to use your body first. You need an emergency procedure.

You need a fire drill.

Think about it. A fire drill is not about understanding the chemical composition of fire. It is not about analyzing why the fire started. It

1

is about knowing exactly where the exits are and how to get out of the building—*fast*.

This book is your Anxiety Fire Drill.

What This Is and What It Is Not

This guide is short. Intentionally so. When you are overwhelmed, you do not need a long lecture on the history of anxiety. You need an actionable checklist.

Let's be clear: This is not a replacement for therapy. It is not a deep exploration of the root causes of your anxiety. It is not a magic cure that promises you will never feel anxious again.

This is a toolkit. It is a first-aid kit for your mind.

It is designed for the moments when you feel the panic rising. For the 3 AM worry sessions. For the sudden dread before a meeting. It is for when you need relief *right now*.

The Approach: Body First, Mind Second

The 7-Minute Reset detailed here is a sequence of five simple, scientifically grounded techniques designed to calm your physiological response, ground your mind in the present reality, and stop the spiral before it escalates.

The core principle is simple: Body First, Mind Second.

We start by using specific techniques to calm the physiological stress response. We manually activate the body's calming mechanisms. Once the physical panic subsides, the thinking brain comes back online. Then, and only then, can we effectively address the anxious thoughts and gain perspective.

The Goal

The goal is not to ensure you never feel anxious again. Anxiety is a normal human emotion. The goal is to equip you with the skills to manage the anxiety effectively when it shows up. It is about recognizing the alarm, realizing it is false, and knowing exactly how to shut it off.

When you know exactly what to do when the alarm goes off, it stops being so terrifying.

These techniques are simple, but they require practice. A fire drill is only effective if you have rehearsed it.

Let's begin the drill.

Robert Duane McDonald

Introduction

It is 3 AM. The room is quiet, but your mind? It's loud. Maybe it started with a thought about that presentation tomorrow. Or perhaps it was a noise downstairs. Or maybe it was nothing at all—just a sudden, jarring realization that you are awake when you should be asleep.

And then it begins.

The heart rate speeds up. A tightness forms in the chest. The thought about the presentation morphs into a certainty that you will fail, lose your job, and end up destitute. Sounds dramatic when you write it down, right? But in the grip of anxiety, these leaps in logic feel entirely real. This is what people mean when they talk about an anxiety spiral. It's not just being nervous. It's a feedback loop where physical sensations create fear, and that fear creates more severe physical sensations.

This book is about interrupting that loop.

We are living in a time often referred to—perhaps dramatically—as the "Age of Anxiety." The pressures are constant. The digital world demands we are always "on." The economic and social landscapes feel uncertain. The numbers back this up. Large-scale studies show that anxiety disorders are among the most common mental health concerns globally (Kessler et al., 2005). It's not just a few people struggling; it's a widespread issue.

But here's the thing about anxiety: much of the suffering doesn't come from the initial worry. It comes from how we react to that worry. We get anxious about being anxious. We panic about the panic. And that, frankly, is where the real trouble starts.

The Promise of the Quick Reset

There is immense value in long-term strategies, therapy, and lifestyle changes. If someone is dealing with debilitating anxiety,

4

professional help is essential. No question about it. But what about the moments in between? What about the sudden surge of panic before a meeting? What about the overwhelming dread that hits on a Sunday evening?

In those moments, you don't need a deep exploration of your past. You need a fire extinguisher. You need a way to bring the nervous system back to baseline, quickly and effectively.

This guide offers exactly that: quick tools to calm the mind and regulate the body in 7 minutes or less. These are not cures. Let's be realistic. They are coping mechanisms. They are techniques grounded in physiology and cognitive behavioral science, designed to stop the spiral before it takes hold.

The goal here isn't to ensure you never feel anxious again. That's impossible, and honestly, unhealthy. Anxiety is a normal human emotion. It's an alarm system. If you see a bear in the woods, you *should* feel anxious. That adrenaline helps you run. The problem occurs when the alarm system goes off because you received an email with the subject line "Quick Question." The alarm is malfunctioning. It's signaling a life-threatening danger when what you are actually facing is mild discomfort or uncertainty.
These resets help you recalibrate the alarm system. They teach you to recognize the difference between a real threat and a perceived one.

Why "Calm Down" Doesn't Work

If you've ever been in the middle of an anxiety spiral and someone told you to "just calm down" or "stop worrying," you know how utterly useless that advice is. It's like telling someone with a broken leg to "just walk normally."

When anxiety takes hold, the rational part of the brain—the prefrontal cortex—starts to go offline. The emotional brain—the limbic system—takes over. In this state, logic is hard to access. You see, you cannot easily think your way out of a feeling state.

Trying to fight the anxiety head-on often makes it worse. When you notice your heart pounding and you think, "Oh no, I'm panicking. I have to stop this right now. If I don't stop, something terrible will happen," you are adding fuel to the fire. You are reinforcing the brain's belief that there is a genuine emergency.

This is a concept known as *secondary disturbance*. The primary disturbance is the initial anxiety about the presentation. The secondary disturbance is your anxiety *about* the anxiety. And guess what? The secondary disturbance is often far worse than the primary one.

People tie themselves in knots trying to eliminate discomfort. They demand certainty in an uncertain world. They believe that they *must* feel comfortable at all times. But this belief? It's irrational. Life is inherently uncomfortable sometimes. Accepting the initial discomfort, without demanding it go away, is the first step to stopping the spiral.

The techniques in this book work because they don't rely on trying to argue with your anxious thoughts while you are in a heightened state. Instead, they focus on two main strategies:

1. **Body-Up Regulation:** Changing your physical state to signal safety to your brain.
2. **Cognitive Interruption:** Shifting your focus away from the internal spiral and grounding you in the present reality.

They are active, not passive. You have to *do* something.

The Anatomy of a Spiral

Let's look closer at how a spiral happens. It usually follows a predictable pattern. Understanding this pattern is crucial because it shows us where we can intervene.

1. **The Trigger:** This can be external (an email, a crowded room) or internal (a random thought, a physical sensation like a skipped heartbeat).
2. **The Perception:** The brain immediately interprets the trigger. If you have a sensitive anxiety system, the interpretation is often "This is dangerous."

3. **The Automatic Thought:** A thought pops up, usually a "What if?" scenario. "What if I faint?" "What if I make a fool of myself?"
4. **The Emotion:** This thought generates a feeling—fear, panic, dread.
5. **The Physical Response:** The body reacts. Adrenaline is released. Heart rate increases. Breathing becomes shallow.
6. **The Misinterpretation:** This is the critical step. The physical symptoms are noticed and misinterpreted as proof that something is terribly wrong. "My heart is pounding—I must be having a heart attack."
7. **The Intensification:** This misinterpretation generates more fear, which generates more physical symptoms. The loop tightens. The spiral accelerates.

The 7-Minute Reset techniques are designed to intervene at steps 5, 6, and 7. They address the physical response directly, help you avoid misinterpretation, and prevent intensification.

Case Example: Mark and the Meeting

Let's consider Mark. He works in marketing and generally enjoys his job. However, he has a deep fear of speaking in front of groups. He is scheduled to give a five-minute update in a team meeting.

The night before, Mark starts to worry. This is the trigger (the upcoming meeting) and the perception (public speaking is dangerous). His automatic thought is: "I'm going to forget what to say, and everyone will think I'm incompetent."

He feels a wave of dread (emotion). His stomach clenches, and he starts sweating (physical response).

Now, here's where the spiral takes hold. Mark notices his physical symptoms. He thinks, "Look how nervous I am already. I can't handle this. When I get in the room tomorrow, I'm going to completely freeze up. I'm going to panic so badly I might have to run out of the room." (Misinterpretation and Intensification).

Mark is no longer just worried about the presentation. He is now terrified of his own anxiety response. He spends the night tossing and turning, visualizing disaster. By the time the meeting arrives, he is exhausted and hyper-alert, making the panic much more likely.

Now, let's imagine Mark had access to these reset tools.

When he noticed his stomach clenching, instead of falling into the "I can't handle this" narrative, he could have recognized it. "Okay, my body is reacting to a perceived threat. This is just adrenaline. It's uncomfortable, but it's not dangerous."

He could then use a physiological technique (like the one we will discuss later) to slow his heart rate. This sends a signal back to the brain that the emergency is over. Once his body is calmer, he could use a cognitive tool (like the "Fact Check") to challenge the thought that everyone will think he's incompetent.

The difference is profound. In the first scenario, Mark is a victim. In the second, he is actively managing his response. The anxiety might not disappear completely—that's not the goal—but it doesn't spiral out of control.

The Role of Acceptance

One of the biggest misconceptions about managing anxiety is that you need to fight it or conquer it. But anxiety is a slippery opponent. The harder you fight, the stronger it seems to get.

A core component of stopping the spiral is *acceptance*. Now, hold on. Acceptance does not mean resignation. It doesn't mean you like feeling anxious. It doesn't mean you give up and let anxiety wash over you.
Acceptance, in this context, means acknowledging the reality of the present moment without judgment. It means saying, "Right now, I am feeling anxious. My heart is racing. My thoughts are swirling. This is where I am."

When you stop demanding that the feeling go away, you stop the secondary disturbance. You stop the anxiety about the anxiety. This often takes the edge off the initial feeling.

Think of it like quicksand. If you fall into quicksand, your instinct is to struggle and fight to get out. But struggling makes you sink faster. The way to survive quicksand is to lie back, spread your weight, and float on the surface. It's counterintuitive, isn't it?

Managing an anxiety spiral is similar. Instead of struggling against the uncomfortable sensations, you acknowledge them and turn your attention to the techniques that will help you "float."

Research in Acceptance and Commitment Therapy (ACT) has shown that willingness to experience uncomfortable internal states, rather than constantly trying to avoid them, is associated with better long-term mental health outcomes (Hayes et al., 2006).

When we try to avoid anxiety, our world becomes smaller. We stop going to social events. We don't take professional opportunities. We organize our lives around avoiding triggers. While this might provide short-term relief, it reinforces the brain's belief that anxiety is dangerous and that we cannot handle it. This sets us up for worse spirals in the future.

The goal is to develop *psychological flexibility*. This is the ability to remain present and take actions that align with your values, even when you are experiencing difficult thoughts and feelings.

Addressing Skepticism

It's natural to be skeptical. If managing anxiety were as simple as a few quick techniques, why is everyone still struggling?

The skepticism usually falls into a few categories.

"This sounds too simple."
The techniques themselves are simple, but implementing them in the heat of the moment? That requires practice. It's like learning any

new skill. Reading about how to swim is different from swimming when you are thrown into the water.

Furthermore, the simplicity is intentional. When you are panicking, you don't have the cognitive resources for complex strategies. You need something you can remember and deploy instantly. We often overcomplicate things, assuming that complex problems require complex solutions. But sometimes, the most effective interventions are the most direct ones.

"I've tried breathing exercises, and they don't work."
Many people have tried generic "deep breathing" when anxious and found it ineffective, or sometimes, it even makes them feel worse. This is often because they are doing it incorrectly or using the wrong type of breathing for their state.

Not all breathing techniques are created equal. The physiological sigh (which we will cover) is fundamentally different from just taking a big breath. It directly targets the mechanism in the lungs responsible for offloading carbon dioxide and signaling calm to the nervous system.

Moreover, breathing is just one tool. If the spiral is primarily cognitive—driven by obsessive thoughts rather than physical panic—a grounding or cognitive diffusion technique might be more effective. This guide provides a toolkit, not a single magic bullet.

"This won't work for my level of anxiety."
It's true that these techniques may not stop a full-blown panic attack that is already at its peak. A panic attack is an intense experience that usually has to run its course (typically peaking within 10 minutes).

However, these tools are designed to be used *before* the peak. They are for the moments when you feel the spiral starting. They can turn what might have been a severe panic attack into a moderate wave of anxiety. They can turn moderate anxiety into mild discomfort.
And even during a severe episode, applying these techniques can help you recover faster. They give you a sense of agency—the

10

feeling that you are not entirely helpless. This sense of agency is crucial.

What to Expect

This guide is structured to be highly practical. We won't spend excessive time on theory. We will focus on the "how-to."

The key to making these resets work is practice. You wouldn't expect to play a piece of music perfectly the first time you try. Similarly, you need to practice these techniques when you are calm, so they become automatic when you are anxious.

When you are calm, your prefrontal cortex is fully engaged. This is the time to learn. When you are anxious, you rely on what you have already learned. By practicing these resets daily, even for just a few minutes, you are building the neural pathways that will support you when you need them most.

The approach taken here is straightforward and action-oriented. It emphasizes that while your feelings are real, your thoughts are not always true. It focuses on what you can control—your actions and your focus—rather than what you cannot control—the uncertainties of life.

It requires a willingness to tolerate discomfort. It requires acknowledging that you might *prefer* to feel calm, but you don't *have* to feel calm to function. You can act even while feeling anxious.
Let's be clear: this is work. But it's work that pays off. By learning to interrupt the anxiety spiral, you are not just reducing suffering in the moment. You are reclaiming your energy and your focus.

The goal is progress, not perfection. There will be times when the spiral happens too fast. That's okay. Every attempt is a learning experience.

Now, let's move on to understanding exactly what happens in your brain and body when anxiety strikes.

Reviewing the Basics

- **Anxiety Spiral:** A feedback loop where physical symptoms increase fear, and fear increases physical symptoms.
- **The Goal:** To interrupt the spiral quickly using targeted techniques, not to eliminate all anxiety.
- **Secondary Disturbance:** Getting anxious about being anxious. This often causes more suffering than the initial worry.
- **Why "Calm Down" Fails:** Anxiety reduces access to the rational brain (prefrontal cortex), making logical arguments ineffective in the moment.
- **Body-Up Regulation:** Changing your physical state to signal safety to your brain.
- **Acceptance:** Acknowledging the present reality (including the anxious feelings) without judgment, rather than fighting it.
- **Practice is Key:** These techniques must be practiced when calm so they can be deployed automatically when anxious.

The "Anxiety Hijack"

If you want to stop an anxiety spiral, you need to know what you're dealing with. You need to understand the mechanisms at play. When anxiety hits hard, it often feels like your brain and body have turned against you. It feels random, chaotic, and overwhelming.

But it's not random. It's actually a highly coordinated, sophisticated survival system doing exactly what it was designed to do. The problem is, it's doing it at the wrong time.

It's like a smoke alarm. A smoke alarm is essential for safety. If there's a fire, you want it to be loud and insistent. But if the alarm goes off every time you make toast, it's not helpful. It's terrifying and disruptive. You end up constantly on edge, anticipating the alarm.

Anxiety works the same way. It's a survival mechanism that has become hypersensitive. It's reacting to "toast" (emails, social situations, uncertainty) as if it were a "fire" (a life-threatening danger).

When this happens, we call it the "Anxiety Hijack" or, more technically, the Amygdala Hijack. Understanding this process is the key to realizing why we can't just "think" our way out of panic and why we must use the body first.

The Two Pathways to Fear

When you encounter a potential threat, your brain processes the information through two different pathways. This is important, so stick with me here.

1. The "Low Road" (The Quick and Dirty Path)

13

This is the rapid response system. Information from your senses (what you see, hear, touch) goes directly to the *thalamus* (the brain's relay station) and then straight to the *amygdala*.

The amygdala is a small structure located deep in the brain. It's the core of the fear center. Its job is simple: scan for danger and activate the alarm if needed. The amygdala doesn't do nuance. It doesn't do rational analysis. It just reacts.

This pathway is incredibly fast. It happens in fractions of a second, before you are even consciously aware of what's going on. This is a survival advantage. If a snake lunges at you, you don't want to spend time analyzing the species. You want to jump back instantly.

When the amygdala senses danger, it immediately triggers the fight-or-flight response.

2. The "High Road" (The Slower, More Accurate Path)

The information also takes a slower route from the thalamus to the *cortex* (the outer layer of the brain, responsible for rational thought, logic, and decision-making), specifically the prefrontal cortex.

The cortex analyzes the situation in more detail. It puts the threat in context. It decides whether the danger is real and whether the amygdala's reaction was justified.

If the cortex determines it was a false alarm (it wasn't a snake, it was just a rope), it sends a signal back to the amygdala to calm down.

The Hijack Explained

In a well-regulated system, the low road and the high road work together. The amygdala provides the rapid warning, and the cortex provides the accurate assessment.

However, in people prone to anxiety spirals, this balance is disrupted. The amygdala is often hypersensitive. It's constantly scanning for threats and reacting to minor stressors as if they were major emergencies.

At the same time, the cortex's ability to calm the amygdala is weakened. It's like having a very loud alarm and a very weak "off" switch.

The "Anxiety Hijack" occurs when the amygdala (low road) activates the alarm, and the cortex (high road) is unable to intervene quickly enough. The emotional brain takes over, and the rational brain is temporarily sidelined.

This is why, in the middle of a panic attack, people struggle to think clearly. Their working memory is impaired. They can't access the logical arguments that might calm them down. The brain is convinced it is fighting for survival.

As neuroscientist Joseph LeDoux, who pioneered the understanding of these pathways, explains, the wiring from the emotional brain to the cognitive brain is stronger than the wiring from the cognitive brain to the emotional brain (LeDoux, 1996). This means it's much easier for emotions to overwhelm thoughts than it is for thoughts to control emotions.

The Fight-or-Flight Response

When the amygdala activates the alarm, it triggers the release of stress hormones, primarily adrenaline (epinephrine) and cortisol.

This cascade of physiological changes is the fight-or-flight response. It's designed to prepare the body to either fight a predator or run away from it.

Let's break down the symptoms and why they happen. Understanding this is crucial because it helps us demystify the sensations of anxiety. They are not signs that you are dying or going crazy; they are signs that your survival system is activated.

Increased Heart Rate and Palpitations:
- *Why it happens:* The heart pumps faster to deliver oxygenated blood to the major muscle groups (arms and legs) so you can fight or run.

- *What it feels like:* Pounding chest, racing heart, sometimes skipped beats.

Rapid, Shallow Breathing (Hyperventilation):
- *Why it happens:* The body tries to take in more oxygen. However, rapid shallow breathing actually disrupts the balance of oxygen and carbon dioxide (CO_2) in the blood.
- *What it feels like:* Shortness of breath, feeling like you can't get enough air, chest tightness.

Dizziness and Lightheadedness:
- *Why it happens:* The disrupted oxygen/CO_2 balance (from hyperventilation) and the rapid changes in blood flow.
- *What it feels like:* Feeling faint, unsteady, dizzy, or spaced out.

Tingling and Numbness:
- *Why it happens:* Also a result of hyperventilation and changes in blood flow to the extremities.
- *What it feels like:* Pins and needles in the hands, feet, or face.

Digestive Issues:
- *Why it happens:* Digestion is not essential for immediate survival. The body shuts it down to divert energy.
- *What it feels like:* Nausea, stomach cramps, or a "pit" in the stomach.

Muscle Tension:
- *Why it happens:* Muscles prime for action. They brace for impact.
- *What it feels like:* Tightness in the neck, shoulders, and jaw. Trembling or shaking.

The Great Deception

Every single one of these symptoms is uncomfortable. Some are downright terrifying. But here is the most important thing to understand: **They are not dangerous.**
They are the appropriate physiological response to perceived danger.

The great deception of anxiety is that it convinces you these symptoms are the actual threat. You forget about the initial trigger (the email, the meeting) and become terrified of the symptoms themselves.

This is where the spiral accelerates. You notice your heart racing and think, "I'm having a heart attack." You feel dizzy and think, "I'm going to faint."

These catastrophic misinterpretations send a new, even stronger signal back to the amygdala: "The danger is real! It's inside me!" The amygdala responds by releasing even more adrenaline. The symptoms intensify.

This is the core mechanism of a panic attack. It's a feedback loop of fear and physical sensations, fueled by catastrophic misinterpretation. Research has consistently shown that this "fear of fear" is a primary driver of panic disorder (Clark, 1986).

Why You Can't "Think" Your Way Out

When you are in the middle of an Anxiety Hijack, the prefrontal cortex is not functioning optimally.

Telling yourself, "It's just anxiety, it's not dangerous," is often ineffective because the amygdala doesn't speak the language of logic. It speaks the language of sensation and action.

Imagine you are in a burning building. The alarm is blaring. Smoke is everywhere. If someone stood next to you and started giving a lecture on the chemical composition of fire, would it calm you down? No. You need to see an exit sign. You need to feel the fresh air.

When you are panicking, you need signals of safety that the amygdala can understand. Logic and reason (the lecture) are not enough. You need to change your physiology (the fresh air).

This is the fundamental principle behind the 7-Minute Reset strategy: **Body First, Mind Second.**
You must address the physiological state before you can effectively engage the cognitive state. You have to manually shut off the alarm before you can assess the situation rationally.

The Importance of Body-Up Regulation

Body-up regulation (also known as bottom-up processing) refers to techniques that use the body to influence the brain.

The autonomic nervous system has two main branches:

1. **The Sympathetic Nervous System (SNS):** The "gas pedal." This is responsible for the fight-or-flight response.
2. **The Parasympathetic Nervous System (PNS):** The "brake pedal." This is responsible for the "rest-and-digest" response.

When anxiety hijacks the system, the SNS is in overdrive, and the PNS is suppressed.

The goal of body-up regulation is to manually activate the PNS to counteract the SNS. We are essentially hacking the nervous system.

One of the most powerful ways to activate the PNS is through the breath. Breathing is unique because it is both automatic (we do it without thinking) and under conscious control (we can change how we breathe). It acts as a bridge.

By changing the pattern of our breath, we can directly influence our heart rate and overall physiological state. For example, long, slow exhales stimulate the *vagus nerve*, a major component of the PNS, which signals the brain to calm down.

Case Example: Sarah and the Fear of Fainting

Let's look at Sarah. She experiences frequent dizziness when she is anxious, particularly in supermarkets. She has a deep fear that she will faint. She has started avoiding supermarkets.

Sarah is experiencing the Anxiety Hijack.

1. **Trigger:** Crowded supermarket.
2. **Amygdala Activation:** The amygdala perceives the crowd as a threat (feeling trapped).
3. **Physiological Response:** Adrenaline is released. Her breathing becomes shallow (hyperventilation).
4. **Symptom:** Dizziness.
5. **Catastrophic Misinterpretation:** Sarah thinks, "I'm dizzy. I'm going to faint right here. It will be humiliating."

6. **Intensification:** This thought terrifies her. More adrenaline is released. The dizziness increases.
7. **Avoidance:** Sarah leaves the supermarket. The relief she feels reinforces the belief that leaving was necessary.

To break this cycle, Sarah needs to understand the mechanism. The dizziness is caused by hyperventilation. It is uncomfortable but unlikely to make her faint. (In fact, anxiety typically raises blood pressure; fainting is caused by a sudden drop).

When the dizziness starts, instead of rushing to the catastrophic interpretation, she needs to intervene at the physiological level.

If she uses a technique to regulate her breathing, she can correct the oxygen/CO_2 imbalance, and the dizziness will subside. This immediately signals safety to the amygdala.

Once the physical symptom is managed, she can then engage her cortex. "I am not fainting. This is just anxiety. I can stay here."

By staying in the situation and managing the symptom, she is teaching the amygdala that the supermarket is safe. This is how the hijack is dismantled.

Preparing for Action

Understanding the Anxiety Hijack is empowering. It shifts the perspective from "Something is wrong with me" to "My survival system is overactive, and I can learn to regulate it."

It explains why traditional approaches focused solely on changing thoughts often fail when anxiety is high.

The key takeaway is this: When the alarm is blaring, your first job is not to figure out why it went off. Your first job is to shut it off.

You shut it off by sending undeniable signals of safety to the brain through the body.

In the next chapters, we will explore the most effective techniques for doing this. We will start with the fastest way known to calm the nervous system using only the breath: The Physiological Sigh.

Understanding the Hijack

- **Anxiety Hijack:** When the brain's fear center (amygdala) activates the alarm, and the rational brain (cortex) cannot intervene effectively.
- **Fight-or-Flight Response:** A cascade of physiological changes (increased heart rate, rapid breathing, dizziness, etc.) designed for survival.
- **Catastrophic Misinterpretation:** The belief that the physical symptoms of anxiety are dangerous (e.g., "I'm having a heart attack"). This fuels the spiral.
- **Body First, Mind Second:** You must address the physiological state before you can effectively engage the cognitive state. Logic doesn't work when the survival system is fully activated.
- **Body-Up Regulation:** Techniques that use the body to influence the brain, primarily by activating the Parasympathetic Nervous System (the "brake pedal").

Reset 1: The Physiological Sigh (1 Minute)

Now we get to the practical stuff. The first tool is the fastest, most effective way to calm your body down when you are acutely anxious or stressed. It is called the *Physiological Sigh*.

This is not just "deep breathing." It is a specific pattern of breathing that mimics a natural process your body already does. You've probably seen it. When someone has been crying intensely and they start to calm down, they often take a shuddering double inhale followed by a long exhale. That's it. That is a physiological sigh. It also happens automatically during sleep to regulate our breathing.

Recent research has shown that consciously deploying the physiological sigh is a powerful tool for immediate stress reduction. It works because it directly targets the autonomic nervous system, activating the parasympathetic (calming) response and dampening the sympathetic (stress) response (Balban et al., 2023).

This technique takes less than a minute, and you can do it anywhere, anytime. It is the first step in the 7-Minute Anxiety Reset because it provides the rapid bottom-up regulation needed to stop the physical panic.

The Science of the Sigh

To understand why this is so effective, we need to briefly look at the mechanics of breathing. It's actually quite fascinating.

Your lungs are made up of millions of tiny air sacs called *alveoli*. These sacs are where the exchange of oxygen and carbon dioxide (CO_2) takes place.

When you are stressed or anxious, your breathing tends to become rapid and shallow. This pattern causes some of the alveoli to collapse. When this happens, the efficiency of gas exchange is reduced. This can lead to an imbalance in the levels of oxygen and CO_2 in your blood.

Rapid, shallow breathing can cause you to offload too much CO_2 too quickly (hyperventilation). This leads to symptoms like dizziness, lightheadedness, and increased anxiety.

The physiological sigh works because it re-inflates the collapsed alveoli. The double inhale is the key. The first inhale fills the lungs partially, and then the second, shorter inhale (a "top-up") forces air into the deflated sacs, popping them open.

When the alveoli are properly inflated, the efficiency of gas exchange is restored.

Furthermore, the long, slow exhale is crucial for activating the parasympathetic nervous system. When you exhale, your diaphragm moves up. By extending the exhale longer than the inhale, you are emphasizing the slowing down phase of the heart rate. This signals to the brain that you are safe and activates the calming response. Slow breathing techniques have long been known to reduce physiological arousal (Jerath et al., 2006).

The physiological sigh combines these two mechanisms—re-inflating the alveoli and activating the parasympathetic nervous system—making it uniquely potent and rapid.

How to Perform the Physiological Sigh

The technique is simple, but the execution matters. It is not the same as just taking a big breath.

Here is the step-by-step guide:

Step 1: The Double Inhale (Through the Nose)
- Take a full, deep inhale through your nose, filling your lungs from the bottom up (feel your belly expand).

22

- Once you feel like your lungs are full, immediately take a second, shorter inhale through your nose (a "top-up"). This second inhale is crucial.

Step 2: The Long Exhale (Through the Mouth)
- Exhale slowly and completely through your mouth. Make the exhale longer than the inhale.
- Try to empty your lungs completely.

The Sequence: Inhale - Inhale (short) - Exhale (long).
That is one cycle.

How Many Repetitions?
Usually, just one to three cycles are enough to significantly reduce acute anxiety and restore a sense of calm. You should feel the effect almost immediately. If you are extremely panicked, you might need up to five times. But start with one.

Common Mistakes and Tips for Success

While the technique is simple, there are a few common mistakes to avoid:

- **Inhaling Through the Mouth:** Try to inhale through your nose if possible. Nasal breathing is generally more calming. However, if your nose is blocked, mouth inhaling is better than nothing.
- **Exhaling Too Quickly:** The exhale should be slow and controlled. Do not force the air out all at once. You can purse your lips (like blowing through a straw) to help control the speed.
- **Forgetting the Second Inhale:** The double inhale is essential. Make sure the second inhale is distinct, even if it is short.
- **Breathing Too High in the Chest:** Try to initiate the breath from your diaphragm (belly breathing).

When to Use the Physiological Sigh

The physiological sigh is versatile. You can use it in any situation where you feel stressed, anxious, or overwhelmed.

- **Before a stressful event:** Before a presentation, an exam, or a difficult conversation.
- **During a stressful event:** While stuck in traffic or when you receive bad news.
- **When you notice physical symptoms:** As soon as you feel your chest tighten or your heart rate increase.

The beauty of the physiological sigh is that it is discreet. You can do it sitting at your desk or in a meeting.

A Case Example: Maria's Overwhelm

Let's look at Maria. She is a working mother juggling a demanding job and two young children.

One evening, Maria is trying to cook dinner while helping her son with homework. The baby starts crying, and the pot on the stove boils over. Maria feels a surge of overwhelm. Her chest tightens, and she feels like she is about to snap.

This is the perfect moment for the physiological sigh. Instead of reacting automatically (by yelling), Maria pauses.

She performs one physiological sigh:

1. Double inhale through the nose: She breathes in deeply, filling her belly, and then takes a quick second inhale.
2. Long exhale through the mouth: She breathes out slowly and completely.

She repeats it one more time.

Immediately, Maria feels a shift. The tension in her chest loosens. Her heart rate slows down. The sense of panic subsides. She is still in the same chaotic situation, but her physiological response to it has changed.

The physiological sigh provided the bottom-up regulation she needed to bring her prefrontal cortex back online. Now she can think clearly and prioritize. This entire intervention took less than 30 seconds.

24

Integrating the Sigh into Your Life

The key to making this work is consistency. Do not just use it as an emergency brake. Use it proactively throughout the day.

Try anchoring the practice to existing habits. For example:

- Do three physiological sighs every time you open your email.
- Do one physiological sigh every time you stop at a red light.

By integrating the sigh into your daily routine, you train your nervous system to return to a state of calm more quickly.

Why This Works When Deep Breathing Fails

You might be thinking, "I've tried deep breathing, and it didn't work." There are reasons why this might be more effective.

1. **It's Faster:** Traditional deep breathing exercises often require several minutes. The physiological sigh works in seconds.
2. **It Addresses Alveolar Collapse:** The double inhale specifically targets the physiological changes that occur during stress.
3. **It Mimics a Natural Process:** Because it is a natural reflex, your body recognizes it and responds readily.

If you have struggled with deep breathing in the past, give this a try. It is a different approach.

In the context of the 7-Minute Anxiety Reset, the physiological sigh is always the first step. It is the quickest way to stop the physical panic and bring your thinking brain back online.

When you feel the anxiety spiral starting, your immediate response should be: Stop. Sigh.

Once you have calmed your body down, you can then move on to the next tool: the 5-4-3-2-1 Grounding Method.

Mastering the Sigh

- **The Technique:** Double inhale through the nose (full inhale followed by a short top-up) and a long, slow exhale through the mouth.
- **The Science:** The double inhale re-inflates the alveoli; the long exhale activates the parasympathetic (calming) nervous system.
- **Deployment:** One to three cycles are usually enough to reduce acute anxiety in seconds.
- **Use It First:** This is the first step. It provides the rapid bottom-up regulation needed to calm the body before addressing the mind.

Reset 2: The 5-4-3-2-1 Grounding Method (2 Minutes)

So you've done the Physiological Sigh. Your heart rate has started to slow down, and the immediate sense of physical panic is beginning to subside. You've interrupted the physiological stress response. But what about the thoughts? Often, even if the body calms down slightly, the mind is still racing, stuck in a loop of worry.

This is where the second tool comes in: The *5-4-3-2-1 Grounding Method*. This technique is designed to pull you out of your head and bring you back to the present moment. It shifts your focus from the internal chaos of your thoughts to the external reality of your environment.

Grounding is crucial because anxiety is almost always future-focused. You are worried about what *might* happen. "What if I fail?" "What if they judge me?" When you are lost in these "what-ifs," you are disconnected from the present moment, where you are actually safe.

The 5-4-3-2-1 method uses your five senses to anchor you to the here and now.

Why Grounding Works: Shifting the Focus

The brain cannot focus on internal thoughts and external sensory input simultaneously with the same intensity. When you are highly anxious, your attention is turned inward.

The 5-4-3-2-1 method works by forcing your brain to switch modes. It gives your brain a specific job to do: find and identify sensory information.

When you consciously focus on what you can see, touch, hear, smell, and taste, you are engaging the parts of your brain responsible

27

for processing sensory information. This pulls resources away from the anxious thoughts.

Furthermore, grounding signals safety to the amygdala. By observing your environment objectively and recognizing that there is no immediate danger, you dampen the stress response. The amygdala realizes that the internal alarm does not match the external reality.

This technique is widely used in various therapeutic approaches, including trauma therapy, because it is effective at bringing people back to the present when they feel overwhelmed (Levine, 2010).

It is a form of mindfulness, but it is more structured and active than traditional meditation. Instead of trying to empty your mind (which is difficult when anxious), you are filling your mind with objective sensory information.

How to Perform the 5-4-3-2-1 Grounding Method

The technique involves identifying a specific number of things in your environment using each of your five senses, in descending order. It takes about two minutes.

Pause and Acknowledge.

Before you start, take a moment to pause and acknowledge that you are feeling anxious. Don't fight it. Just notice it.

Step 1: FIVE Things You Can SEE
- Look around and identify five distinct things.
- Say the name of each item out loud (if possible) or in your mind.
- Be specific and detailed. Instead of just "chair," think "brown wooden chair with a blue cushion."
- Look for small details—a crack in the wall, a pattern on the floor.

Step 2: FOUR Things You Can TOUCH

- Identify four distinct things you can physically feel.

- Reach out and touch them, or focus on the sensation of things already in contact with your body (like your clothes or the chair you are sitting on).

- Notice the texture, temperature, weight, and shape.

Step 3: THREE Things You Can HEAR
- Tune in to the sounds and identify three distinct sounds.

- Close your eyes if it helps.

- Listen for sounds you might normally tune out—the hum of the air conditioner, the ticking of a clock, the sound of traffic outside.

Step 4: TWO Things You Can SMELL
- Identify two distinct smells.

- This can be challenging. You can move around to find smells, or focus on subtle scents (like coffee from the breakroom or hand sanitizer).

- *Tip:* If you cannot smell anything, identify your two favorite smells instead.

Step 5: ONE Thing You Can TASTE
- Identify one thing you can taste.

- Focus on the taste in your mouth right now. If you have a drink or gum, focus on that.

- *Tip:* If you cannot taste anything, identify your favorite taste. Finish with a Deep Breath.

After completing the sequence, take another deep breath (or a physiological sigh) and notice how you feel.

Tips for Making It Work

The effectiveness of this method depends on how engaged you are.

- **Be Specific and Detailed:** The more detail you notice, the more your brain has to work, and the more effectively it pulls you out of the anxious spiral. Don't rush.

- **Say It Out Loud:** If the situation allows, saying the name of the items out loud enhances the effect. It engages the language centers of your brain.
- **Move Your Body:** When identifying things to touch, physically reach out. When looking, move your head and eyes. This physical movement can also help discharge anxious energy.
- **If You Get Distracted, Start Over:** Your mind will wander. That is normal. When you notice you are distracted, gently bring your attention back.

A Case Example: David's Social Anxiety

Let's look at David. He is at a networking event and feels overwhelmed by social anxiety. He is convinced everyone is judging him. His mind is racing with thoughts like "I don't belong here."

David steps aside and uses the 5-4-3-2-1 method.

5 See: He identifies the pattern on the carpet, a woman in a red dress, the condensation on his water glass, a painting on the wall, and a waiter carrying a tray.
4 Touch: He focuses on the coolness of the glass in his hand, the stiffness of his collar, the pressure of his shoes on the floor, and the texture of the wall next to him.
3 Hear: He tunes into the chatter of the crowd, the clinking of glasses, and the background music.
2 Smell: He notices the smell of perfume and the aroma of the food being served.
1 Taste: He takes a sip of water.
After completing the exercise, David feels more present. His focus has shifted from his internal worries to the external environment. He realizes that no one is actually watching him. It allowed him to stay at the event and engage.

Adapting the Technique

The 5-4-3-2-1 method is flexible.

- **When Driving:** Keep your eyes on the road. Identify things related to driving (speedometer, road sign). Focus on physical sensations (steering wheel, seat). Identify sounds (engine, radio).

- **When Lying in Bed:** If it is dark, identify shapes or shadows. Focus on the sensation of the blanket and mattress. Listen for sounds in the house.

Why Sensory Detail Matters

It is important to emphasize the role of detail. If you just quickly list "chair, table, floor, wall, window," it won't be very effective. The goal is to engage your brain fully in the task of observation.

When you look for specific details, you are forcing your brain to work harder. This provides a stronger interruption of the anxious thoughts.

Combining the Sigh and the Grounding

The physiological sigh and the 5-4-3-2-1 method work together. The sigh provides the physiological reset; the grounding method provides the cognitive reset.

The sequence is:

1. Physiological Sigh (1-3 repetitions) - Calm the body.

2. 5-4-3-2-1 Grounding Method - Anchor the mind.

This sequence takes about three minutes. At the end of it, your prefrontal cortex should be back online, allowing you to think clearly.

Moving to the Next Step

Once you have calmed your body and anchored your mind, you are ready for the next phase: engaging your thinking brain.

Now you can start to address the anxious thoughts that triggered the spiral in the first place. You can evaluate them rationally.

In the next chapter, we will introduce the third tool: the Fact Check. This will help you distinguish between facts and fears.

Grounding in Reality

- **Anchor to the Present:** The 5-4-3-2-1 Method pulls you out of anxious thoughts and brings you back to the present moment, where you are safe.
- **Engage Your Senses:** The technique uses your five senses (See, Touch, Hear, Smell, Taste) to shift your focus from internal chaos to external reality.
- **Be Detailed:** The more detail you notice, the more effective the technique.
- **Combine with the Sigh:** Use the physiological sigh first to calm the body, then the 5-4-3-2-1 method to anchor the mind.

Reset 3: The "Fact Check" (CBT Technique) (2 Minutes)

By this point in the reset process, you have deployed the Physiological Sigh and the 5-4-3-2-1 Grounding Method. You have interrupted the immediate panic. The physiological hijack is over.

However, the underlying thoughts that triggered the anxiety might still be there, lingering. If you do not address these thoughts, the anxiety is likely to return.

This is where the third tool comes in: The "Fact Check." This technique is derived from Cognitive Behavioral Therapy (CBT), a highly effective approach to treating anxiety. CBT is based on the idea that our thoughts, feelings, and behaviors are interconnected, and that by changing our thoughts, we can change how we feel (Beck, 2011).

The Fact Check is a rapid way to evaluate your anxious thoughts rationally. It helps you distinguish between facts and fears, reality and imagination.

The Power of Irrational Beliefs

Anxiety is rarely caused by the situation itself. It is caused by your interpretation of the situation. When you feel anxious, it is usually because you are holding onto irrational beliefs about the situation.

These beliefs often fall into a few common categories, known as *cognitive distortions*:

- **Catastrophizing (Awfulizing):** Assuming the worst possible outcome. "If I mess up this presentation, I will lose my job and my career will be over."
- **Mind Reading:** Assuming you know what others are thinking. "Everyone in the room thinks I'm incompetent."

33

- **Fortune Telling:** Predicting the future negatively, without evidence. "I know I'm going to fail."
- **All-or-Nothing Thinking:** Seeing things in extremes. "If I'm not perfect, I'm a failure."
- **Should Statements:** Having rigid rules about how you and others should behave. "I shouldn't feel anxious."

These distortions are automatic. They pop into your head without effort. And if you accept them as facts, they trigger the anxiety response.

The Fact Check is designed to interrupt these automatic thoughts and examine them critically. It's about putting your thoughts on trial and demanding evidence.

How to Perform the Fact Check

The Fact Check involves asking yourself a series of questions. It takes about two minutes.

Step 1: Identify the Anxious Thought
- First, identify the specific thought causing the anxiety. What are you telling yourself?

- Pinpoint the most distressing thought. It often starts with "What if..."

- *Example:* "I'm going to bomb this interview and never get a job."

Step 2: Ask: Is This Thought a Fact or an Opinion/Fear?
- This is the core question. Is the thought an objective fact, verifiable by evidence? Or is it an opinion, a feeling, or a prediction?

- A *fact*: "The interview is at 10 AM."
- A *fear*: "I'm going to bomb the interview."
- In almost all cases, the anxious thought is not a fact. Recognizing this immediately reduces its power.

Step 3: Demand Evidence: What Supports This Thought?
- Now, put the thought on trial. What evidence do you have that this thought is true?

34

- Look for objective facts, not feelings.

- *Example:* "I stuttered in my last interview." (Fact)

Step 4: Demand Evidence: What Contradicts This Thought?
- Now, look for evidence that contradicts the thought.

- *Example:* "I prepared thoroughly." "I have the qualifications for the job." "I've had successful interviews in the past."

Step 5: Identify the Cognitive Distortion
- Based on the evidence, identify the distortion. Are you catastrophizing? Mind reading?

- Giving the distortion a name helps you recognize it as an irrational pattern.

- *Example:* "I am fortune telling and catastrophizing."

Step 6: Reframe the Thought: What is a More Realistic View?
- Finally, develop a balanced view based on the evidence.

- This is not about positive thinking. It is about accurate thinking.

- *Example:* "I might feel nervous, and it might not go perfectly. But I am prepared. Even if I don't get this job, it doesn't mean I will never get a job."

This new, realistic thought will not eliminate anxiety completely, but it will reduce it significantly. It shifts the perspective from "I am doomed" to "This is challenging, but I can handle it."

A Case Example: Ben's Health Anxiety

Let's look at Ben. He has a headache and immediately worries it might be a brain tumor. His anxiety escalates.

Ben uses the Fact Check.

Step 1: Identify the Thought: "This headache means I have a brain tumor."
Step 2: Fact or Fear? It is a fear. The fact is "I have a headache."
Step 3: Evidence Supporting?
- "I have a headache." (No objective evidence linking this specific headache to a tumor.)

Step 4: Evidence Contradicting?

- "I didn't sleep well."

- "I've been stressed."

- "Headaches are common."

- "I had a checkup recently and was healthy."

Step 5: Identify the Distortion: Catastrophizing.

Step 6: Reframe the Thought: "I have a headache, likely due to stress or lack of sleep. While it's possible it could be serious, it is highly unlikely. If it persists, I will call my doctor."

This process shifts Ben's focus from the irrational fear to rational management.

The "Thought vs. Evidence" Worksheet

To make the Fact Check process more concrete, you can use a simple worksheet mentally or on paper.

Anxious Thought	Evidence For	Evidence Against	Realistic Reframe
(Catastrophic thought)	(Objective facts supporting)	(Objective facts contradicting)	(Balanced, evidence-based thought)

Using this structure forces you to confront the evidence (or lack thereof).

Common Challenges and How to Overcome Them

When you start using the Fact Check, you might encounter challenges:

- **"But it feels true!"** Anxious thoughts feel real because they are accompanied by strong emotions. Remember that feelings are not facts. Acknowledge the feeling, but evaluate the thought objectively.

- **"But what if the worst happens?"** It is possible. The Fact Check is not about guaranteeing a positive outcome. It is about evaluating the probability. Most of the time, the catastrophic outcome is highly improbable. And even if it does happen, the Fact Check helps you realize that you can cope.
- **Difficulty Finding Evidence Against:** When anxious, you might struggle to find contradictory evidence. Anxiety biases your attention towards negative information. You might need to actively search for positive evidence.
- **Automatic Thoughts are Persistent:** Anxious thoughts are habitual. They will not disappear overnight. You will need to practice the Fact Check repeatedly.

The Shift from "What If" to "What Is"

Anxiety is driven by "What if." The Fact Check shifts your focus to "What is."

- "What if I fail?" (Anxiety)
- "What is the evidence that I will fail?" (Fact Check)

This shift from future prediction to present reality is crucial. You can deal with what is happening right now. You cannot deal with the infinite possibilities of the future.

By practicing the Fact Check regularly, you become more aware of your cognitive distortions. You start to recognize the patterns. Eventually, it becomes automatic.

This leads to a profound shift. You realize that you are not your thoughts. You are the observer of your thoughts. And you have the power to choose which thoughts to believe.

Challenging the Narrative

- **Challenge Your Thoughts:** Anxiety is fueled by cognitive distortions. Do not accept your anxious thoughts as facts.
- **Identify the Thought:** Pinpoint the specific thought causing the anxiety.

37

- **Demand Evidence:** Ask: "Is this a fact or a fear?" "Where is the proof?" Evaluate the evidence for and against.
- **Reframe Realistically:** Develop a balanced view based on the evidence. This is about accuracy, not positivity.
- **Practice:** The Fact Check is a skill that requires practice. The more you use it, the more automatic it becomes.

Reset 4: The "Zoom Out" Perspective Shift (1 Minute)

You have calmed your body, anchored your mind, and challenged your catastrophic thoughts. You are feeling more in control. But you might still feel stressed by the situation. The problem might still seem significant.

This is where the fourth tool comes in: The "Zoom Out" Perspective Shift. This technique is designed to help you gain perspective and reduce the perceived importance of the stressor. It interrupts the tendency to magnify the significance of the stressor and helps you see the bigger picture.

When you are anxious, you develop tunnel vision, focusing exclusively on the immediate threat. The stressor fills your entire mental landscape. It feels like the most important thing in the world.

The Zoom Out deliberately broadens your perspective. It is like zooming out on a map, shifting from the street view to the city view, and then to the global view.

The Tyranny of the Immediate

Our brains are wired to prioritize immediate threats. This is a survival mechanism. If a lion is chasing you, you need to focus entirely on escaping.

However, in modern life, this tendency leads to chronic stress. We treat every deadline, every social interaction, every minor setback as if it were life-or-death. We magnify the importance of the present moment and forget the bigger picture.

This narrow focus increases the pressure. If we believe that the outcome of this one event determines our entire future, we are bound to feel anxious.

The Zoom Out interrupts this process by introducing a sense of scale. It reminds us that most of the things we worry about are not actually that important in the long run. This perspective shift is a core component of philosophical traditions like Stoicism that emphasize emotional resilience (Aurelius, trans. 2002).

How to Perform the Zoom Out

The Zoom Out involves asking yourself a series of questions that progressively broaden your perspective in time and space. It takes about one minute.

Step 1: Acknowledge the Stressor
- First, acknowledge the situation causing stress. Define the problem.

- *Example:* "I am stressed about the feedback on my project."

Step 2: The Temporal Zoom Out (Time Perspective)
- Now, ask yourself:
    - **"Will this matter in 5 days?"** Will you still be worrying about this specific feedback next week? (Maybe, but less intensely.)
    - **"Will this matter in 5 months?"** Will this one project still be a major focus? (Probably not.)
    - **"Will this matter in 5 years?"** Will you even remember this feedback? (Highly unlikely.)
- This "5-5-5 Rule" helps you put the stressor in the context of your life span. It highlights the temporary nature of the problem.

Step 3: The Spatial Zoom Out (Space Perspective)
- Now, ask yourself:
    - **"How important is this compared to other challenges I have faced?"** Have you overcome more difficult situations? (Almost certainly yes.)
    - **"How important is this compared to the challenges other people are facing?"** Think about people dealing with serious illness or war. Does your problem seem as significant? (Usually not.)

- o **"How important is this in the grand scheme of the universe?"** Imagine looking down from space. How small does your problem seem? (Infinitesimally small.)
- This sequence reduces the sense of self-importance and isolation that often accompanies anxiety.

Step 4: Re-evaluate the Significance
- Finally, re-evaluate the significance of the stressor.

- *Example:* "This feedback is important for my current project, but it is not a measure of my worth, nor will it determine my entire life. It is just one data point."

This process rapidly reduces the perceived threat level. It doesn't eliminate the problem, but it shrinks it down to a manageable size.

A Case Example: Lisa's Traffic Jam Frustration

Let's look at Lisa. She is stuck in a massive traffic jam and is going to be late for a meeting. She feels angry, stressed, and helpless.

Lisa uses the Zoom Out.

Step 1: Acknowledge the Stressor: "I am stuck in traffic and will be late."
Step 2: Temporal Zoom Out:
- **5 Days?** Will being late matter next week? Maybe slightly, but the meeting will be over.
- **5 Months?** No, the meeting will be forgotten.
- **5 Years?** Absolutely not.

Step 3: Spatial Zoom Out:
- **Compared to past challenges?** I have dealt with much worse things (e.g., illness).
- **Compared to others' challenges?** Being stuck in traffic is an inconvenience, not a tragedy.
- **Grand scheme?** This traffic jam is utterly insignificant.

Step 4: Re-evaluate: "Being late is frustrating, but not a catastrophe. I will apologize when I arrive. Right now, there is nothing I can do about the traffic, so I might as well relax."

This helps Lisa shift from anger and panic to acceptance and calm.

The Power of "Compared to What?"

A key component of the Zoom Out is the comparison. We tend to evaluate our situation in isolation. By asking "Compared to what?", we introduce a sense of scale.

This is not about minimizing your feelings. It is about recognizing that your interpretation of the problem is subjective and can be changed.

Avoiding Nihilism and Minimization

It is important to use this technique carefully to avoid falling into nihilism (the belief that nothing matters) or minimizing real problems.

The goal is not to convince yourself that your life is meaningless. The goal is a balanced perspective.

Some things *do* matter. If you are dealing with a serious crisis, the Zoom Out might not be as helpful, or it might need to be adapted. It should not be used to avoid dealing with the problem.
The Zoom Out is most effective for the everyday stressors that we tend to blow out of proportion—the deadlines, the social awkwardness, the minor setbacks.

The Role of Acceptance

The Zoom Out also fosters acceptance. When you realize that the situation is temporary and relatively insignificant, it becomes easier to accept it as it is, rather than resisting it.

Anxiety often stems from non-acceptance. "This shouldn't be happening."

The Zoom Out helps you shift to: "This is happening. It is temporary. I can handle it."

Acceptance means acknowledging reality as it is, so you can respond effectively.

The "Overview Effect" in Daily Life

Astronauts who have seen the Earth from space often report a profound shift in perspective known as the *Overview Effect*. When they see the Earth as a small, fragile ball, their personal concerns seem insignificant (White, 2014).

The Zoom Out technique allows you to experience a mini version of this. By mentally zooming out, you can achieve a similar sense of calm and clarity.

Moving to Action

Once you have gained perspective, you are ready for the final step: taking action.

Anxiety often leads to paralysis. The final tool, the One Next Step, is designed to break the overwhelm and move you forward.

Gaining Perspective

- **Broaden Your View:** Anxiety narrows your focus. The Zoom Out broadens your perspective in time and space.
- **Use the 5-5-5 Rule:** Ask: "Will this matter in 5 days? 5 months? 5 years?" This highlights the temporary nature of the problem.
- **Use the Spatial Zoom Out:** Ask: "How important is this compared to past challenges? In the grand scheme of the universe?"
- **Re-evaluate:** Shrink the stressor down to a manageable size.
- **Foster Acceptance:** The Zoom Out helps you accept the situation as it is, shifting the mindset from "catastrophe" to "temporary and manageable."

Reset 5: The "One Next Step" Method (1 Minute)

We have reached the final step. You have systematically addressed the physiological, cognitive, and emotional components of the anxiety response. You are calm, grounded, rational, and have perspective. Now what?

Now, it is time to take action.

Anxiety thrives on inaction. When we feel overwhelmed, we tend to freeze. We get stuck in a loop of rumination, unable to move forward. This paralysis increases the anxiety, because the problem remains unsolved and the pressure builds.

The fifth tool is the "One Next Step" Method. This is designed to break the overwhelm and move you into action. It is about identifying the smallest, most immediate, and most manageable action you can take right now.

It shifts the focus from "How do I feel?" to "What do I do?"

The Paralysis of Overwhelm

When faced with a large or threatening situation, our brains tend to perceive it as a single, insurmountable obstacle. We see the mountain, not the path.

This perception of overwhelm triggers the stress response, which impairs the prefrontal cortex—the part responsible for planning. So, when we most need to think clearly, our cognitive abilities are compromised.

We get stuck in "analysis paralysis." We overthink, analyzing every possible outcome. We search for the perfect solution, and when we cannot find it, we do nothing.

44

The One Next Step method interrupts this cycle by shrinking the scope of the problem. It shifts the focus from the daunting outcome to the immediate process.

The Power of Small Wins

The rationale is based on the psychology of motivation. Research shows that the most effective way to achieve large goals is to break them down into small, achievable steps and focus on consistent progress (Clear, 2018).

Small wins build momentum and self-efficacy (the belief in your ability to succeed). When you complete a small task, your brain releases a small amount of dopamine (the reward neurotransmitter). This makes you feel good and motivates you to take the next step.

Furthermore, taking action directly counteracts the helplessness that accompanies anxiety. When you act, you assert control. You shift from passive victim to active agent.

How to Identify the One Next Step

The method involves asking a simple question: **"What is the smallest, most immediate action I can take right now to move forward?"**
The key words are *smallest*, *immediate*, and *action*.
- **Smallest:** The step should be so small it feels easy. If it feels daunting, break it down further.
- **Immediate:** Something you can do right now, with the resources you have.
- **Action:** A concrete behavior, not a thought. "Think about the problem" is not an action. "Write down three possible solutions" is an action.
Here is the guide:

Step 1: Define the Situation (Briefly)
- Quickly summarize the problem. Do not get bogged down in analysis.
- *Example:* "I am overwhelmed by this project deadline."

Step 2: Ask the Key Question

- "What is the One Next Step I can take right now?"

- *Example:* "Open the project document."

Step 3: If Necessary, Break It Down Further

- If the identified step feels overwhelming, break it down further.

- *Example:* If "Open the document" feels too hard, the next step might be "Turn on the computer."

Step 4: Take the Action (Immediately)

- Do it immediately, without hesitation.

- Do not think about the entire project. Focus solely on this one small action.

Step 5: Acknowledge the Progress

- Acknowledge that you have taken a step forward.

Step 6: Repeat the Process

- Once the first step is complete, ask the question again: "What is the next step?"

This method gradually builds momentum and moves you through the task, one step at a time.

A Case Example: Alex's Exam Anxiety

Alex has a major exam tomorrow and hasn't studied enough. He is paralyzed by anxiety, convinced he will fail. Instead of studying, he is procrastinating.

Alex uses the One Next Step method.

Step 1: Define the Situation: "I am overwhelmed by studying."
Step 2: Ask the Key Question: "What is the One Next Step?"

- His mind says: "Study the entire textbook." (Too big.)

- He breaks it down: "Study Chapter 1." (Still too big.)

- He breaks it down further: "Open the textbook to Chapter 1." (Manageable.)

Step 3: Take the Action: Alex opens the textbook.

Step 4: Acknowledge: "Okay, I've started."
Step 5: Repeat: "What is the next step?"
- "Read the first paragraph." (Manageable.)

By focusing on one small step, Alex bypasses the overwhelm. He might not cover everything, but he makes progress, which reduces his anxiety.

The 15-Minute Sprint

Another way to implement this is the "15-Minute Sprint." This is useful when you feel strong resistance.

Commit to working on the task for just 15 minutes. Tell yourself: "I will work on this for 15 minutes, and then I can stop if I want to."

This small commitment reduces the perceived difficulty and makes it easier to start. Often, once you start, the momentum carries you forward.

Action Precedes Motivation

A common misconception is that we need to feel motivated before we can act. We wait for inspiration or for the anxiety to subside.

But in reality, it often works the other way around: Action precedes motivation.

When you take action, you generate motivation. You see progress, you feel accomplishment, and this fuels your desire to continue.

The One Next Step method leverages this. It does not require you to feel motivated or calm. It asks you to act *despite* the anxiety.

Dealing with Resistance

You might encounter resistance. Your mind might come up with excuses. "I don't have enough time." "I need to plan more first."

This resistance is often a manifestation of anxiety or perfectionism.

When you encounter resistance, acknowledge it, but do not let it stop you. Ask: "Despite the resistance, what is the smallest action I can take?"

If the resistance is strong, make the step ridiculously small. If "Write the report" feels impossible, try "Write one sentence."

The size of the step does not matter. What matters is the direction of the movement.

The Importance of "Good Enough"

It is important to adopt a mindset of "good enough." Perfectionism is the enemy of action. If you wait for the perfect conditions, you will never start.

The goal is progress, not perfection. The One Next Step does not have to be the ideal step. It just has to be a step forward.

By accepting "good enough," you reduce the pressure and the fear of failure. You give yourself permission to act imperfectly.

The 7-Minute Anxiety Reset prepares you to face challenges with clarity and resilience. Once you have completed the reset, you are ready to engage with the world.

Moving Forward

- **Break the Overwhelm:** Anxiety leads to paralysis. The One Next Step method breaks overwhelm by shrinking the scope and focusing on immediate action.
- **Identify the Smallest Action:** Ask: "What is the smallest, most immediate action I can take right now?" Break it down until it feels easy.
- **Build Momentum:** Small actions lead to progress, which builds momentum. Action precedes motivation.
- **Use the 15-Minute Sprint:** If you feel resistance, commit to just 15 minutes.

- **Adopt a "Good Enough" Mindset:** Focus on progress, not perfection.

Creating Your Personal Reset Routine

You now have five powerful tools in your anxiety first-aid kit. Individually, each tool can help. But when combined, they provide a comprehensive system for interrupting the anxiety spiral.

This chapter is about creating your personal reset routine. It is about integrating these tools into your life so you can use them effectively when you need them most.

The 7-Minute Anxiety Reset is a flexible framework you can adapt. The goal is a routine that works for you and that you can deploy automatically.

Reviewing the Five Tools

Let's briefly review the tools and their roles:

1. **The Physiological Sigh (1 Minute):** Bottom-up regulation. Calms the body.
2. **The 5-4-3-2-1 Grounding Method (2 Minutes):** Anchors the mind to the present.
3. **The Fact Check (2 Minutes):** Top-down regulation. Challenges catastrophic thoughts.
4. **The Zoom Out (1 Minute):** Top-down regulation. Gains perspective.
5. **The One Next Step (1 Minute):** Action-oriented. Breaks overwhelm.

The sequence is intentional. We start with the body to stop the panic and bring the thinking brain online. Then we engage the mind. Finally, we move into action.

Body -> Mind -> Action.

The Full 7-Minute Reset Sequence

Here is the full sequence in a checklist format. Keep this handy.

The 7-Minute Anxiety Reset Checklist
[ ] Step 1: Calm the Body (1 Minute)
  . • Perform 1-3 Physiological Sighs: Double inhale (nose), long exhale (mouth).

[ ] Step 2: Anchor the Mind (2 Minutes)
  • Use 5-4-3-2-1 Grounding: 5 See, 4 Touch, 3 Hear, 2 Smell, 1 Taste.

[ ] Step 3: Challenge the Thoughts (2 Minutes)
  • Use the Fact Check: Identify thought. Fact or Fear? Demand evidence. Reframe.

[ ] Step 4: Gain Perspective (1 Minute)
  • Use the Zoom Out: Will this matter in 5 days? 5 months? 5 years?

[ ] Step 5: Take Action (1 Minute)
  • Use the One Next Step: What is the smallest action right now? Do it.

Adapting the Routine to Your Needs

You might not always have the time or need for all five tools.

The 1-Minute Mini-Reset (For Mild Anxiety)
  • **Physiological Sigh (30 seconds):** 1-3 sighs.
  • **One Next Step (30 seconds):** Identify and take immediate action.

The 3-Minute Emergency Reset (For Moderate Anxiety)
  • **Physiological Sigh (30 seconds):** Calm the body.
  • **5-4-3-2-1 Grounding (2 minutes):** Anchor the mind.
  • **One Next Step (30 seconds):** Take action.

The Cognitive Reset (For Worry)
If your anxiety is primarily cognitive (worry, rumination) and less physiological.

  • **Fact Check (2 minutes):** Challenge the thoughts.
  • **Zoom Out (1 minute):** Gain perspective.

Identifying Your "Go-To" Tools

As you practice, you might find that some tools resonate more than others. Identify your "go-to" tools—the ones that work best for you.

Experiment and observe their effects. Pay attention to which tools provide the most immediate relief.

The Importance of Practice (When Calm)

I cannot emphasize this enough: **You must practice these tools when you are calm.**
If the first time you try this is in the middle of a panic attack, it will be much harder. Your thinking brain will be offline.

It is like a fire drill. You practice the procedure when there is no fire so that when a real fire occurs, you know exactly what to do.

- **Daily Practice:** Dedicate 7 minutes each day to practicing the full sequence.
- **Situational Practice:** Practice in low-stakes situations. Practice the sigh while waiting in line, or the 5-4-3-2-1 method while commuting.
- **Visualization:** Mentally rehearse the sequence. Imagine yourself feeling anxious and successfully using the tools.

The goal is to make the reset routine a habit.

Recognizing the Early Warning Signs

To use the routine effectively, you need to recognize the early warning signs. Anxiety usually builds up gradually.

If you can catch it early, the reset routine will be much more effective.

- **Physical Signs:** Increased muscle tension, shallow breathing, slightly increased heart rate, restlessness.
- **Cognitive Signs:** Increased worry, difficulty concentrating, negative thinking patterns.
- **Behavioral Signs:** Avoidance, procrastination, fidgeting.

As soon as you notice these signs, deploy the routine. Do not wait.

Troubleshooting Common Problems

Problem: "I can't remember the steps when I'm anxious."

Solution: Practice more when calm. Keep a checklist handy. If you cannot remember the full sequence, just use the one tool you remember (e.g., the sigh).

Problem: "The tools are not working."

Solution: Check your execution. Are you performing the techniques correctly? Give it time. The routine reduces anxiety, but might not eliminate it completely. If the anxiety is very high, you might need to repeat the sequence.

Problem: "I forget to use the tools."

Solution: Anchor the habit to existing habits (e.g., every time you check your phone). Set reminders. Practice recognizing early warning signs.

A Case Example: Creating James's Routine

James, a software developer, often felt anxious before meetings.

James's Practice Routine:
- He practiced the full 7-Minute Reset every morning.
- He kept a checklist on a sticky note on his monitor.

James's "Go-To" Tools:
- He found the Physiological Sigh most effective for physical symptoms.
- He found the Fact Check most helpful for catastrophic thoughts.

James's Adapted Routine:
- **Before Meetings (Mini-Reset):** 5 minutes before, he would do three Physiological Sighs and a quick Fact Check.
- **When Noticing Tension (Proactive):** Whenever he noticed tension in his shoulders, he would immediately do a Physiological Sigh.

By creating a personalized routine, James managed his anxiety effectively.

The Long-Term Goal: Building Resilience

The 7-Minute Anxiety Reset is not just a quick fix. It is a tool for building long-term emotional resilience—the ability to bounce back from stress.

Every time you use the routine, you are training your nervous system to return to calm more quickly. You are strengthening the neural pathways associated with emotional regulation.

Over time, your amygdala becomes less reactive, and your prefrontal cortex becomes stronger.

The 7-Minute Anxiety Reset is an investment in your mental health. It is a skill that will serve you for life.

Your Personalized Plan

- **Master the Sequence:** Understand the role of each tool and the intentional sequence (Body -> Mind -> Action).
- **Adapt the Routine:** Adapt the routine using Mini-Resets and identifying your "go-to" tools.
- **Practice When Calm:** Practice regularly when calm to make them automatic.
- **Recognize Early Signs:** Learn to recognize early warning signs and deploy the reset immediately.
- **Build Resilience:** View the routine as a tool for building long-term resilience, not just a quick fix.

Prevention: Micro-habits for a Calmer Mind

The 7-Minute Reset manages anxiety when it arises. But what if you could reduce its frequency and intensity in the first place?

This chapter is about prevention. It is about cultivating simple daily habits—*micro-habits*—that support a calmer mind.
Anxiety is deeply connected to your physical health. Sleep, nutrition, movement, and stress all play a significant role.

By making small, consistent changes, you can significantly reduce your vulnerability. These are small, manageable actions you can sustain.

The Concept of Baseline Anxiety

Think of your anxiety level like a thermometer. There is a baseline level. When you encounter a stressor, the level rises. If your baseline is already high, it takes very little stress to push you into overwhelm.

If your baseline is low, you can handle significant stress. You have a buffer zone.

The goal of these micro-habits is to lower your baseline anxiety.

Here are three key areas to focus on: physical regulation, cognitive regulation, and environmental regulation.

Micro-Habit 1: Physical Regulation

Your brain and body are connected. If your body is stressed, your mind will be stressed.

Hydration: The Simplest Calming Tool

Dehydration is a common contributor to anxiety. Even mild dehydration can increase cortisol (stress hormone) and cause symptoms that mimic anxiety (e.g., increased heart rate, dizziness).

The Micro-Habit: Drink a glass of water upon waking, and sip consistently throughout the day.

Nutrition: Balancing Blood Sugar

Diets high in sugar and refined carbohydrates cause spikes and crashes in blood sugar. These fluctuations can trigger adrenaline and cortisol, leading to anxiety and irritability.

The Micro-Habit: Focus on balanced meals with protein, healthy fats, and complex carbohydrates to stabilize blood sugar.
- **Actionable Tip:** Start your day with a protein-rich breakfast.

Limiting Caffeine and Alcohol

Caffeine is a stimulant that increases adrenaline, which can exacerbate anxiety and interfere with sleep.

Alcohol is a depressant that can initially feel relaxing, but it disrupts sleep and can increase anxiety in the long run (the rebound effect or "hangxiety").

The Micro-Habit: Be mindful of consumption.
- **Caffeine:** Limit intake and avoid it in the afternoon/evening.
- **Alcohol:** Limit intake and avoid using it as a coping mechanism.

Movement: Discharging Stress Energy

Physical activity is highly effective for reducing anxiety. Exercise burns off excess adrenaline, releases endorphins (mood boosters), and improves sleep. Regular exercise can be as effective as medication for mild to moderate anxiety (Sharma et al., 2006).

Even mild activity like walking or yoga makes a difference.

The Micro-Habit: Incorporate movement daily.
- **Actionable Tip:** Go for a 15-30 minute walk every day. Stand up and stretch every hour.

Micro-Habit 2: Cognitive Regulation

A rested mind is a calmer mind.

Prioritizing Sleep: The Foundation of Resilience

Sleep deprivation is a major contributor. When sleep-deprived, your amygdala (threat detector) becomes more reactive, and your prefrontal cortex (emotional regulation) becomes less effective.

The Micro-Habit: Aim for 7-9 hours of quality sleep. Establish a consistent sleep schedule.
- **Actionable Tip:** Create a relaxing bedtime routine (reading, warm bath) to wind down.

Mindfulness and Meditation:

Mindfulness is paying attention to the present moment, without judgment. It helps you become aware of your thoughts without getting caught up in them.

The Micro-Habit: Practice mindfulness throughout the day.
- **Actionable Tip:** Take "mindful moments." When drinking coffee, focus on the aroma and taste. Dedicate 5-10 minutes daily to meditation (guided app or breath focus).

Journaling: Processing Thoughts and Emotions

Journaling is a powerful tool for processing emotions and reducing rumination. Writing down worries can help externalize them.

The Micro-Habit: Spend 5-10 minutes daily journaling.
- **Actionable Tip:** Try "expressive writing," where you write freely about your feelings without worrying about structure (Pennebaker & Smyth, 2016).

Gratitude: Shifting the Focus

Gratitude is acknowledging the good things. It shifts your focus from what is lacking to what is positive.

The Micro-Habit: Practice gratitude daily.
- **Actionable Tip:** Every evening, write down three specific things you are grateful for.

Micro-Habit 3: Environmental Regulation

Your environment plays a significant role.

Digital Boundaries: Managing Information Overload

Constant connection and information overload lead to chronic stress. Constant exposure to negative news and social comparison fuels anxiety.

The Micro-Habit: Set boundaries around technology use.
- **Actionable Tip:** Take regular breaks (e.g., phone-free hours morning/evening). Be selective about information consumption. Turn off non-essential notifications.

Personal Boundaries: Protecting Your Energy

Lack of boundaries leads to overwhelm and burnout. Learning to say no and protecting your energy is crucial.

The Micro-Habit: Practice setting boundaries.
- **Actionable Tip:** Start small. Say no to one small request this week that you would normally accept out of obligation.

Connection: The Power of Support

Social connection is a fundamental need and a powerful buffer against stress. Isolation can exacerbate anxiety.

The Micro-Habit: Nurture your relationships.
- **Actionable Tip:** Schedule regular time with friends/family. Reach out and share your feelings.

The Power of Consistency

The key is consistency. Small actions repeated consistently lead to significant changes.

Do not try to implement all these habits at once. Start small. Choose one or two habits and focus on integrating them.

Start with a version of the habit that is easy. Instead of 30 minutes of meditation, commit to 2 minutes.

Be patient and compassionate. The goal is progress, not perfection.

Prevention and intervention work together. The micro-habits lower your baseline anxiety, and the 7-Minute Reset provides a tool to manage acute episodes.

Building a Calmer Baseline

- **Lower Baseline Anxiety:** Micro-habits lower your baseline anxiety, creating a buffer against stress.
- **Physical Regulation:** Focus on hydration, balanced nutrition, limiting caffeine/alcohol, and regular movement.
- **Cognitive Regulation:** Prioritize sleep, practice mindfulness, journal, and practice gratitude.
- **Environmental Regulation:** Set digital and personal boundaries, and nurture social connections.
- **Start Small:** Choose one or two habits. Consistency is key.

Conclusion & When to Seek More Help

We have reached the end of this guide. You now have a comprehensive toolkit for managing anxiety. The 7-Minute Anxiety Reset provides a structured, scientifically grounded approach to interrupting the anxiety spiral.

The journey is not about eliminating anxiety completely. It is about developing the skills to navigate life with more ease and confidence.

The Core Principles of the Reset

The 7-Minute Anxiety Reset is based on a few core principles:

Anxiety is Physiological

Anxiety is a full-body experience. Recognizing it is physiological helps reduce shame. It is not a weakness; it is biology.

Bottom-Up Regulation is Key

When acutely anxious, the thinking brain goes offline. You must use your body (breathing, grounding) to calm the physiological response first.

Thoughts are Not Facts

Anxiety is fueled by irrational beliefs. You do not have to believe everything you think. By challenging your thoughts (Fact Check), you can break the cycle of catastrophic thinking.

Perspective Shifts the Experience

The perceived importance of a stressor is subjective. By broadening your perspective (Zoom Out), you can reduce emotional reactivity.

Action Breaks the Paralysis

Anxiety thrives on inaction. By breaking down tasks (One Next Step), you can overcome paralysis and regain agency.

Consistency is Crucial

Managing anxiety is a skill requiring practice. Consistent practice trains your nervous system to be more resilient.

A Lifelong Practice

Managing anxiety is a lifelong practice. There will be times when you feel overwhelmed. That is normal.

The key is self-compassion and persistence. Be kind to yourself when you struggle. Acknowledge your progress.

Every time you use the 7-Minute Anxiety Reset, you are strengthening your ability to regulate your emotions.

When These Tools Are Not Enough

The 7-Minute Anxiety Reset is powerful, but it is not a substitute for professional help. If you are experiencing severe or persistent anxiety that interferes with your daily life, seek support.

Self-help tools are effective for mild to moderate anxiety. But anxiety disorders are complex and often require professional treatment.

Signs You Should Seek Professional Help

How do you know when to seek help?

- **Intensity and Duration:** Anxiety is severe, persistent, and overwhelming, lasting for weeks or months, and not improving with self-help.
- **Impairment in Daily Functioning:** Anxiety significantly interferes with work, relationships, or daily activities.
- **Panic Attacks:** You experience recurrent, unexpected panic attacks.

- **Avoidance Behaviors:** You go to great lengths to avoid triggers, restricting your life.
- **Physical Symptoms:** Anxiety is accompanied by severe physical symptoms (chronic pain, insomnia).
- **Rumination and Worry:** You are constantly worrying and cannot stop the cycle of negative thoughts.
- **Co-occurring Conditions:** You are also experiencing symptoms of depression or substance abuse.
- **Thoughts of Self-Harm or Suicide:** If you experience these thoughts, seek immediate professional help. Call a crisis hotline or go to the emergency room.

Types of Professional Help Available

The most effective treatment often involves therapy and, in some cases, medication.

Therapy

Therapy provides a safe space to explore causes, develop skills, and change patterns.

- **Cognitive Behavioral Therapy (CBT):** The gold standard. Focuses on identifying and challenging negative thought patterns.
- **Exposure Therapy:** Gradually exposing yourself to feared situations in a safe environment to learn coping.
- **Acceptance and Commitment Therapy (ACT):** Focuses on accepting difficult thoughts rather than controlling them, and committing to valued actions.

Medication

Medication can help reduce the severity of symptoms, especially combined with therapy.

- **Antidepressants (SSRIs and SNRIs):** Often the first-line treatment, balancing neurotransmitters.
- **Anti-Anxiety Medications (Benzodiazepines):** Provide rapid relief but are generally short-term due to habit-forming potential.

Medication decisions must be made with a qualified healthcare professional.

How to Find Help

Finding the right professional takes effort.

- **Primary Care Physician:** Can provide referrals and rule out medical conditions.
- **Insurance Provider:** Provides a list of in-network professionals.
- **Online Directories:** Websites like Psychology Today or the Anxiety and Depression Association of America (ADAA) offer directories.
- **Employee Assistance Programs (EAP):** May offer confidential counseling.

It is important to find a therapist you feel comfortable with and who has experience treating anxiety.

A Final Word of Encouragement

Managing anxiety is a journey. It requires courage, commitment, and self-compassion.

You have taken the first step by seeking tools. You have the capacity to change your relationship with anxiety.

The 7-Minute Anxiety Reset provides a roadmap. Practice the tools consistently. Cultivate the habits. Seek help if needed.

Remember that you are not alone. Anxiety is common, and there is hope.

You have the power to stop the spiral and live a life not dictated by fear. Start now. Breathe. Ground. Fact-check. Zoom out. Act.

You can do this.

The Path Ahead

- **Embrace the Principles:** Remember the core principles: physiological basis, bottom-up regulation, thoughts are not facts, power of perspective, and importance of action.

- **Commit to Practice:** View anxiety management as a lifelong practice requiring consistency and self-compassion.
- **Recognize Limits:** Self-help tools are not a substitute for professional help when anxiety is severe.
- **Know When to Seek Help:** Be aware of the signs (impairment, panic attacks, avoidance, self-harm).
- **Take Action:** If struggling, seek professional help. You do not have to do this alone.

References

Aurelius, M. (2002). *Meditations* (G. Hays, Trans.). Modern Library. (Original work published ca. 161–180 CE)

Balban, M. Y., Neri, E., Kogon, M. M., Weed, L., Nouriani, B., Jo, B., Holl, G., Zeitzer, J. M., Spiegel, D., & Huberman, A. D. (2023). Brief structured respiration practices enhance mood and reduce physiological arousal. *Cell Reports Medicine, 4*(1), 100895. https://doi.org/10.1016/j.xcrm.2022.100895

Beck, J. S. (2011). *Cognitive behavior therapy: Basics and beyond* (2nd ed.). Guilford Press.

Clark, D. M. (1986). A cognitive approach to panic. *Behaviour Research and Therapy, 24*(4), 461–470. https://doi.org/10.1016/0005-7967(86)90011-2

Clear, J. (2018). *Atomic habits: An easy & proven way to build good habits & break bad ones.* Penguin Random House.

Hayes, S. C., Luoma, J. B., Bond, F. W., Masuda, A., & Lillis, J. (2006). Acceptance and commitment therapy: Model, processes and outcomes. *Behaviour Research and Therapy, 44*(1), 1–25. https://doi.org/10.1016/j.brat.2005.06.006

Jerath, R., Edry, J. W., Barnes, V. A., & Jerath, V. (2006). Physiology of long pranayamic breathing: Neural respiratory elements may provide a mechanism that explains how slow deep breathing shifts the autonomic nervous system. *Medical Hypotheses, 67*(3), 566–571. https://doi.org/10.1016/j.mehy.2006.03.042

Kessler, R. C., Berglund, P., Demler, O., Jin, R., Merikangas, K. R., & Walters, E. E. (2005). Lifetime prevalence and age-of-onset distributions of DSM-IV disorders in the National Comorbidity

Survey Replication. *Archives of General Psychiatry, 62*(6), 593–602. https://doi.org/10.1001/archpsyc.62.6.593

LeDoux, J. E. (1996). *The emotional brain: The mysterious underpinnings of emotional life.* Simon & Schuster.

Levine, P. A. (2010). *In an unspoken voice: How the body releases trauma and restores goodness.* North Atlantic Books.

Pennebaker, J. W., & Smyth, J. M. (2016). *Opening up by writing it down: How expressive writing improves health and eases emotional pain.* Guilford Press.

Sharma, A., Madaan, V., & Petty, F. D. (2006). Exercise for mental health. *Primary Care Companion to the Journal of Clinical Psychiatry, 8*(2), 106. https://doi.org/10.4088/pcc.v08n0208a

White, F. (2014). *The overview effect: Space exploration and human evolution* (3rd ed.). American Institute of Aeronautics and Astronautics.

9 781923 604261